Can I tell you about Eczema?

A guide for friends, family and professionals

JULIE COLLIER

Illustrated by Apsley

Foreword by Margaret Cox

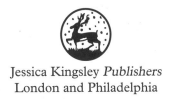

Jessica Kingsley *Publishers*
London and Philadelphia

First published in 2015
by Jessica Kingsley Publishers
73 Collier Street
London N1 9BE, UK
and
400 Market Street, Suite 400
Philadelphia, PA 19106, USA

www.jkp.com

Library of Congress Cataloging in Publication Data
A CIP catalog record for this book is available from the Library of Congress

British Library Cataloguing in Publication Data
A CIP catalogue record for this book is available from the British Library

ISBN 978 1 84905 564 2
eISBN 978 0 85700 999 9

Printed and bound in Great Britain
by Bell and Bain Ltd, Glasgow

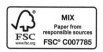

MIX
Paper from
responsible sources
FSC
www.fsc.org
FSC® C007785

Can I tell you about Eczema?

Can I tell you about...?

The "Can I tell you about...?" series offers simple introductions to a range of limiting conditions and other issues that affect our lives. Friendly characters invite readers to learn about their experiences, the challenges they face, and how they would like to be helped and supported. These books serve as excellent starting points for family and classroom discussions.

Other subjects covered in the "Can I tell you about...?" series

ADHD

Adoption

Anxiety

Asperger Syndrome

Asthma

Autism

Cerebral Palsy

Dementia

Depression

Diabetes (Type 1)

Dyslexia

Dyspraxia

Eating Disorders

Epilepsy

ME/Chronic Fatigue Syndrome

Nut Allergy

OCD

Parkinson's Disease

Pathological Demand Avoidance Syndrome

Selective Mutism

Stammering/Stuttering

Stroke

Tourette Syndrome

To my children, Michael and Chloe, and in memory of my dad, David Richards, with love.

Acknowledgements

I would like to thank my mum, Pauline Richards, for her help and support with my Eczema as I was growing up and now, as an adult. My long-suffering husband, Andy! My daughter, Chloe, who has had Eczema since she was four months old and now manages it really well.

Mal Leicester for asking me to write the foreword to her book *Can I tell you about Tourette Syndrome?* and for inspiring me to write a book myself. Lucy at JKP, thanks for the nurturing and support and, most of all, your patience. Margaret Cox, Chief Executive of the National Eczema Society and the dermatology nurse Julie Van Onselen, thank you for reading through the book and for making some really good suggestions. You are all wonderful!

Contents

Foreword

If you are reading this book the chances are that you have Eczema in your family. If so, you don't need me to tell you that Eczema is not just a bit of dry skin. It is a truly challenging condition to live with. Alas not everyone understands that.

Julie and her daughter understand the trials of Eczema all too well. More importantly, they have a wealth of experience and practical tips to share with other families who are struggling to manage this – all too literally – irritating and on occasions, hugely frustrating condition.

With one in five schoolchildren in the UK now developing Eczema, it is sad that one of the most frequent messages we hear at the National Eczema Society is from parents who feel desperately alone, who imagine they are the only ones finding it hard to keep the Eczema under control and who despair as their children scratch their skin, sometimes until it bleeds.

For this reason I am so glad that Julie has written this book. Eczema is, unfortunately, a very common condition, and if your child has Eczema and you sometimes find it hard to control, you are certainly *not* alone. And while Eczema can indeed be hard to manage at times, as Julie demonstrates it does not have to destroy family life.

Eczema is a highly visible condition and society tends to judge us on how we look. Because so many things in our environment can set off an Eczema flare, lifestyle adjustments can be a necessity. For a child, looking different from and being treated differently to their peers can be very uncomfortable.

This excellent book explains what Eczema is in language a child can understand, which will make it easier for them to live a full and confident life. It is well suited to being read at home together with parents and caregivers, and would also be a great help in schools and community groups to make sure that children who do not have Eczema do have an understanding of what the condition entails.

Eczema may be challenging but it does not have to control our lives. By telling their story in such an accessible and engaging manner, Julie and Helen are helping millions of children living with Eczema, and I am truly grateful to them.

Margaret Cox
Chief Executive, National Eczema Society

Introduction

Can I tell you about Eczema? is written for families, friends and professionals and it aims to help everyone to gain a greater understanding of Atopic Eczema in children. Atopic Eczema (sometimes known as Atopic Dermatitis) describes an inherited form of Eczema that is linked to the atopic gene (that also is responsible for Asthma and Hay fever). It is the main type of Eczema seen in children, and while there are other types of Eczema seen in children and adults, this book will focus on Atopic Eczema, which will be referred to from this point onwards as "Eczema".

- It describes what Eczema is and what it's like to live with. It looks at possible triggers and current treatments.

- Parents will be able to read it with their children and will gain insight into how Eczema may affect their child.

- Teachers can use the book to increase their knowledge and for peer awareness in the classroom. Teachers will also be able to draw upon the useful tips to help the child to cope with their Eczema in school and to do their best in lessons.

- Others will learn how best to support their friend with Eczema.

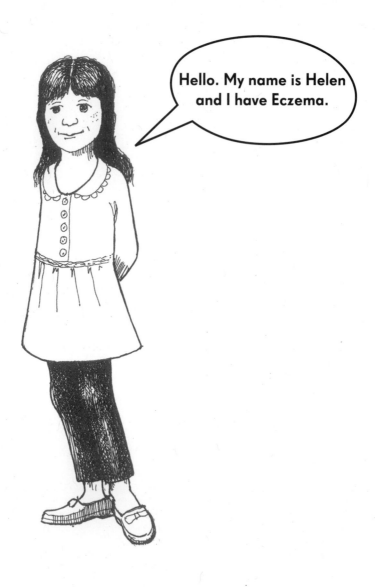

"I have had Eczema since I was a few months old. I would like to tell you about living with Eczema, so that others can feel supported and understood too."

"Some days you might not be able to tell I have anything wrong with my skin and other days it looks really red and sore and you might catch me scratching!

When my skin is very bad, I try to hide it as much as I can with long-sleeved tops and trousers and some days I just don't want to go out. However, as I am getting older I have realised that it doesn't really matter how it looks, as family and friends all know about my Eczema and so I am much more relaxed about it. If I meet new people when it's bad, I tell them I have Eczema and answer any questions they might have.

How Eczema feels has always been the worst thing for me, especially if I have something to do, like homework, a nice place to visit or even if I need to sleep. I start to feel hotter than usual and I get really itchy and very irritable and I find it very hard to concentrate on anything but the parts of my skin that are getting hotter and pricklier by the minute and I just have to *scratch*. Scratching feels really good for a second or two, as it stops the dreadful itch, but then it really hurts and I know I have made my skin worse. Sometimes I scratch so hard that I break the skin and make it bleed and weep (water). You can read about things that can help later in the book. "

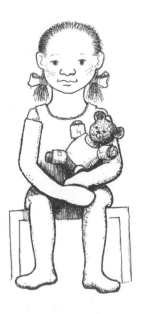

"Sometimes the itching and scratching got so bad that Mum had to bandage my arms and legs with cool wet bandages to help calm down my skin so that I could relax and get to sleep. Not everyone needs bandages/wraps, but talk to your doctor if you think they may help you."

"I have had Eczema since I was a few months old. My mum remembers wrapping me in a towel when I'd had a bath and I started to scratch my tummy really hard.

I don't remember too much about my Eczema when I was very young, but we have lots of pictures with my skin looking really red and sore and I am wearing wet-wrap bandages in lots of the photographs too.

My mum has had quite severe Eczema all of her life and my granddad had it too. This meant that there was a good chance that I might also get Eczema. My older brother doesn't get Eczema, but he gets Hay fever, which you will read about later in the book, as it is linked with Eczema and also Asthma too."

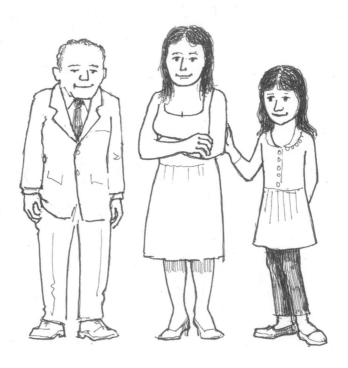

"My mum and granddad have quite bad
Eczema and my cousin has it too. At least
we all understand what it feels like, although
we still tell each other off for scratching!"

"When I was younger my skin used to be so hot and itchy all of the time. I would have to scratch to ease the dreadful itch, but then my skin would get redder, bleed and weep (water) and I would get so sore and very upset. My skin would dry out, get scabby and would often crack and bleed again. The soreness or the itch would often keep me awake or wake me up in the night and I wouldn't be able to sleep for hours. My clothes and bed sheets would be covered in cream and my blood when I had a bad night.

It sometimes feels like I have really bad sunburn all over, from head to toe, and then that thousands of biting ants are running all over me!

Mum says that most of the time Eczema can interrupt daily life but you get used to the routine (e.g. putting cream on) and you learn how to deal with it. However, there have been many days, sometimes weeks, when life has had to have been put on hold for a while whilst the severe flare-ups have been brought under control.

I have never been admitted to hospital with my Eczema, but Mum had to go in several times for intensive treatment, both when she was a child and as an adult."

Ants crawling on your skin

Restlessness

Sleeplessness

Rash

Infections

Watering

Scratching

Tiredness

Treatment

Red

Avoidance

Weeping

Bleeding

Inflammation

Swollen

Stiffness

ITCHY

Raw

Pain

Irritable

HOT

Tears

Cracked

"My Eczema can range from being very good to very bad and it can change quite quickly.

A lot of people may have quite mild Eczema and it is common to only have it on the skin on the inside of the elbows and behind the knees.

Others, like me, can have Eczema covering their whole body and face, including their head and ears too!

Affected skin can look very red, inflamed and dry and scaly. It can look wet when it is weeping or bleeding and scabby too. Little blisters can develop on your hands and feet.

When it is very bad, it can limit your movement, make you feel very stiff and make it difficult to even hold a pencil.

Eczema can affect your sleep, so you may feel very tired and sometimes it can make you feel quite unwell.

When infected, skin can look swollen, red and more angry than usual, it may also weep and may have a yellow crusty appearance. The infection (the bacteria in the skin causing a problem) can make you feel unwell, but don't worry as nobody can catch the infection from you. There is more information about infections on page 29."

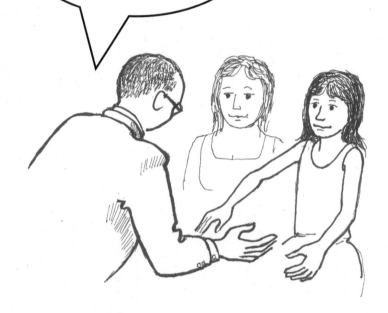

"My mum took me to see the doctor."

"A doctor (GP) or other health-care person will look at your skin and ask your parents/carers about any family history. They will ask you what it feels like and how it affects you. They will be able to treat your Eczema, although sometimes they will need to refer you to a specialist skin doctor, called a dermatologist.

They may prescribe treatments and suggest other ways that you can manage your Eczema. They may want to see you at regular intervals for a while to check up on how the treatments are working and to change them if necessary.

Sometimes your health visitor or nurse may be able to offer support and information too."

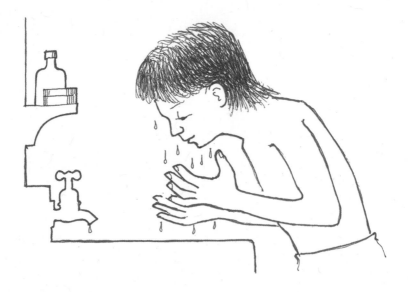

"I wash and shower using the emollients prescribed by my doctor. They help to keep my skin clean and moisturised."

SOAP, DETERGENTS AND PERFUMES

"Soap can dry out the skin of people with Eczema. Anything that contains detergent and perfume also generally makes Eczema worse, as they irritate the skin. This includes all bubble baths and cosmetic wash products.

I always use my emollients or Eczema wash products as soap substitutes, as they work just as well as soap at cleansing my skin, but without the bubbles."

OVERHEATING AND TEMPERATURE CHANGES

"Radiators and gas fires can overheat my skin. Playing sports and any exercise can make me feel hot and itchy too. Eczema can also get worse or better depending on the time of the year, and can often flare when the temperature changes between indoors and outdoors.

I try to keep my bedroom cool at night (about 18°C) and use a fan if I am still too hot. I use a light duvet and I sometimes take an ice pack, wrapped in a cotton pillowcase, and put it on my hot and itchy patches. This helps me to stop scratching and to get to sleep more quickly. I wear cool clothing when doing sports and sip cool water. Sometimes I need a little break to cool down and apply some cream and then I can join in again."

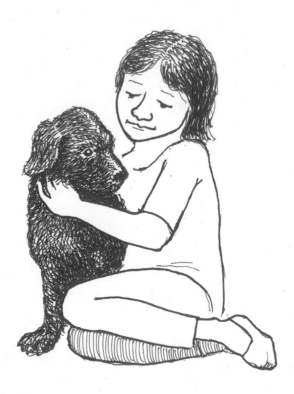

"I am allergic to lots of animals, such as cats, rabbits and horses. While I am allergic to a lot of dogs, we did some research and found a breed that doesn't shed their fur. We still have to keep her clean and her fur cut short though."

ANIMALS

"People with Eczema are usually allergic to all furry animals. We had a rabbit, but he lived outside in his hutch and run and I took antihistamines before I played with him and always washed my hands afterwards.

I have Asthma as well as Eczema and horses can make both really flare up.

After many years of nagging Mum and Dad for a dog and after they had done lots of research and we had spent some time with the breed, we finally got Ria who doesn't shed her fur. Both Mum and I are fine with her, but we have to keep her clipped and washed regularly.

I try to avoid animals that affect my skin wherever possible. If you are thinking of getting a pet for your home, always spend some time with it before making a decision and do some research into how particular breeds affect people with allergies."

FOOD

"Certain foods can cause an allergic reaction and make Eczema flare up. Food is more likely to be a problem for children with Eczema who are less than two years of age, although it is not unheard of in older children and adults. Sometimes the allergic reaction can happen straight after eating, so you know to avoid that food. But other times the reaction may not show up for a while so you cannot be sure what food has caused it. It is important to get any food allergies diagnosed, and to ensure that diets are always used in conjunction with other treatments.

My doctor helped by carrying out some tests to identify some of the foods that I may be allergic to. Some I have to avoid and some I just have to limit."

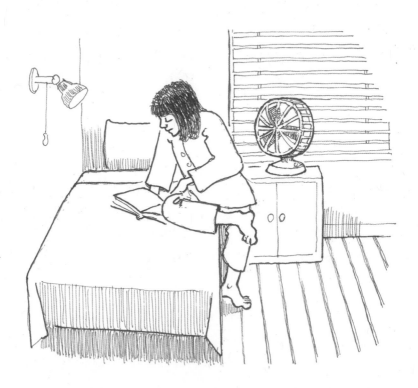

"I wear cotton and try to stay as cool as I can, especially at night."

CLOTHING

"Some fabrics, such as wool, are really itchy and some man-made materials can affect my skin too. I wear 100 per cent cotton clothes wherever possible and use cotton bed linen too. I always take a 100 per cent cotton sheet from home whenever I go for a sleepover. I use a feather-free pillow and duvet too. When I was younger I used specialist seam-free cotton and silk sleep suits, as well as seam-free pyjamas."

WASHING POWDERS

"Biological washing powders/liquids and fabric softeners can sometimes irritate Eczema, causing a flare-up. It is good to use hot washes (to remove grease and house dust mites) and rinse clothes well – use an extra rinse cycle to remove all washing powder/liquid.

My mum only uses non-biological washing powder and never uses fabric conditioner. She says this is because they might irritate my skin and make it worse."

DUST

"Dust and house dust mites can make Eczema worse.

We have chosen to have wooden floors in our house and blinds at many windows instead of curtains. This helps us to reduce the amount of dust. We vacuum and damp dust; (using a damp cloth) regularly to keep the dust down too.

When I was younger, Mum used to wash my soft toys on a hot wash or would put them in a bag in the freezer to kill any dust mites."

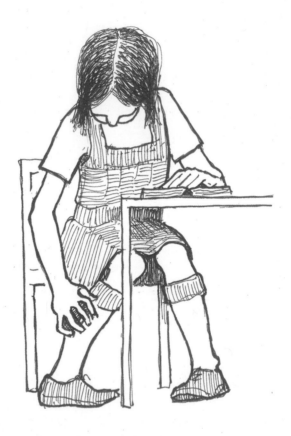

"If I get too hot or stressed at school, I scratch my arms or legs. They bleed and weep and sometimes my socks stick to my legs and I have to soak them off in the bath when I get home."

STRESS

"Sometimes people with Eczema find their skin can become itchier when they are stressed or anxious.

I always talk to my parents or teachers when I feel stressed or worried. Sometimes doing something completely different for a while to take my mind off things can help and I find that listening to music or going for a walk with the dog can really help me."

INFECTION

"Eczema can become infected, as when the protective skin layer is damaged the skin is at risk of infection from bacteria, yeasts and viruses. Therefore skin that is sore, raw and broken can easily become infected.

If I have a cold or a sore throat my Eczema often gets worse. I can easily get an infection in the skin where I have scratched and sometimes my glands swell up too. I know when my skin might be infected as it gets more red and sore and sometimes becomes wet and weepy with yellow crusts. Mum takes me to the doctor as soon as I have any signs of infection in my skin or elsewhere, as it can make me quite poorly quite quickly."

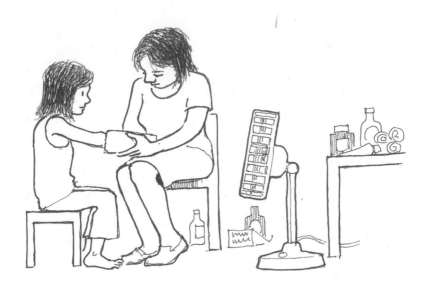

"When I was younger and my Eczema was very bad, Mum used to bath me using bath oil. She would then pat my skin dry very carefully and apply lots of greasy ointments. She would then apply wet-wrap bandages under my pyjamas and give me antihistamines to help me sleep."

"Who can prescribe these treatments? Doctors and nurses (GPs, dermatologists and dermatology nurses at hospitals and clinics). You can also buy some of them over the counter; ask at your local chemist.

Emollients are special moisturisers that help to keep the skin supple and feeling less dry and itchy and much more comfortable. They are also used for washing to replace soap.

It is very important to keep the skin as moisturised as possible by applying creams or ointments at least twice a day or more if needed. This helps to reduce the dryness and the itch by repairing the skin's barrier, stopping water loss, which helps to lock in the skin's own moisture."

CREAMS VERSUS OINTMENTS VERSUS LOTIONS

"A cream is usually white in colour and quite cooling to apply, and an ointment is usually quite see-through and greasy to touch. For extremely dry and itchy skin, an ointment is likely to work better, but may make you feel warmer. There are also some lotions available, which are very light and soak in very quickly. The most important thing is to try different creams, ointments and lotions to find out what suits you the best. Remember that sometimes you may need different ones to use at different times of the day; or you may prefer to use just the one that suits you and your skin. Use them daily; you often need to apply several times a day, whenever your skin feels dry and itchy."

OTHER TREATMENTS

"You can read more about other treatments at the back of the book."

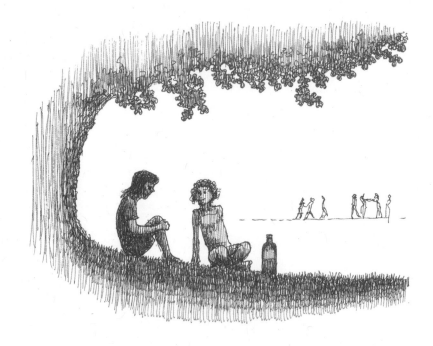

"I head for the shade in the playground and drink cold water to keep me nice and cool."

"Like lots of other health conditions, Eczema can affect your self-esteem and self-confidence (how you feel about yourself). Learning more about it and talking to others about your condition can really help with this. It helps if family members and friends can learn all they can about Eczema too, and ask how they can help. If you are feeling down about your skin, try to think about what is good about yourself and also what you are good at and what you enjoy doing.

I love going on family holidays and sometimes take a friend along. By the end of the holiday my Eczema is usually a lot better, but at the beginning it can be a real struggle. I love to splash about in the sea but the salt water really stings at first and I end up in tears. I put cream on but then the sand sticks to it and sometimes I stay in the caravan or apartment for a while to give my skin a chance to heal up. Mum always takes all of my creams on holiday, so we have them handy if my skin flares up."

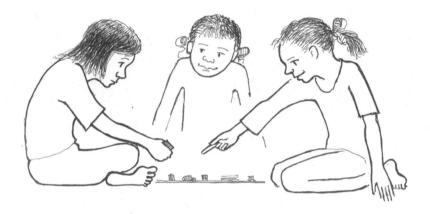

"I love to have friends around to
play games at my house."

"My closest friends all know about my skin and although Eczema is with me every day and I do talk about it I try not to complain too much!

I can remember being called scabby and I felt upset for a short while, and then told myself that I have Eczema and I am a nice person and would never call anyone a name. I felt sorry for the person for being so mean.

On days when my skin is really bad, I don't go out to play. Sometimes I feel too tired and irritable and will need to apply creams quite often. I sometimes stay in my pyjamas, so that it's easier to apply lots of creams without spoiling my good clothes. I sometimes ask friends to come around to my house, so that I can stay in my pyjamas and feel comfy and relaxed. I always make the most of my good days and spend as much time as I can with my friends and family.

Brothers and sisters can feel quite left out when parents or carers are spending more time treating the child with Eczema. I sometimes feel fed up that I have Eczema and they don't, but this doesn't last for long."

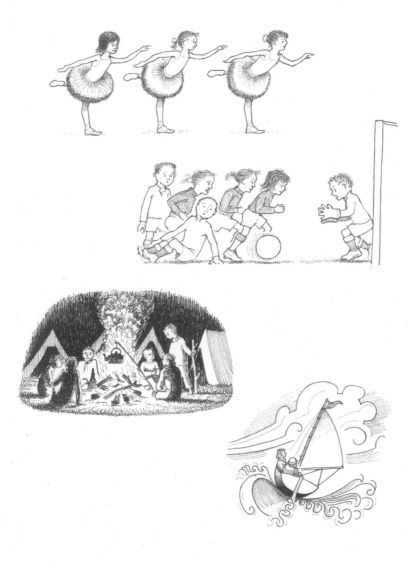

"I enjoy lots of hobbies, including ballet and I go to my local Sea Scouts, where I have lots of friends and we go camping, canoeing, sailing, rock climbing and play all sorts of games."

"Despite having had Eczema all my life, I have lots of lovely friends and some great hobbies. There are always times when I can't join in some of the activities but sometimes I just need to make adjustments so that I can take part.

Chlorine can make me itch and dry out my skin, but I have had swimming lessons for years. I just make sure I shower really well afterwards and put some cream on straight away.

I have been in Sea Scouts for many years and take part in all sorts of activities. I go camping regularly and we play lots of sports. We do lots of water sports in the summer, including sailing, canoeing and rowing. I make sure I wear a T-shirt under my wetsuit and put cream on when I need to. I have missed quite a few sessions because of my Eczema, but I have really enjoyed it when I go. I have represented my group at football matches and sailing competitions too.

I have friends around for sleepovers and they invite me back too. They see how I have to treat my skin and it helps them to understand more."

What is Eczema? The facts

- The word "Eczema" comes from the Greek word meaning "to boil", which is often how having Eczema feels!

- Eczema is a genetic condition, which means it can run in your family and you may have someone else in your family who has it. However, it is a complex immunological condition, and it can be triggered by many things in our environment.

- Atopic Eczema is a very common skin condition with up to 1 in 5 children and 1 in 12 adults affected in the UK. It is also known as Atopic Dermatitis.[1]

- There are several types of Eczema; the most common type is Atopic and an estimated 30 million people in the USA have it.[2]

- Atopic Eczema can affect boys and girls equally.

- About one-third of children with Atopic Eczema will also have Asthma and/or Hay fever as the same atopic gene responsible for Eczema is also responsible for Asthma, Hay fever and some food allergies.

- There is a defect in the skin's barrier which means that when you have Eczema, your skin may not produce enough fat or oil and is less able to retain water, so this plays a part in Eczema development, as the protective skin barrier is not as good as it should be.

---

1   National Eczema Society. "What is Eczema?" available at www.eczema.org/what-is-eczema, accessed on 14 January 2015.

2   National Eczema Society. "Eczema", available at http://nationaleczema.org/eczema, accessed on 14 January 2015.

- The skin of people with Eczema looks red and inflamed and will be itchy. The itch means you want to scratch and this usually makes things worse, as it sets off an "itch–scratch" cycle.

- When Eczema is flaring, skin can become very sore and it can crack, weep and bleed. It is usually very dry and scaly too.

- People with Eczema are more likely to get skin infections and infections can make the skin much worse and sometimes make you feel very unwell too.

- Eczema is definitely not catching.

- Eczema usually starts in the first 18 months and half will grow out of it by the age of 5 and up to 95 per cent by the age of 15. A small percentage will still grow out of it in adulthood. The outlook is not affected by the severity or family history. Flare ups in adults who have apparently grown out of it, can often be controlled with the right treatment.

How Eczema affects school and how school can help

Eczema doesn't always bother people at school. For me, it can be quite difficult at times and sometimes I have to have days off school, as my skin has been so bad. There are things that school can do to help my Eczema:

- If the sun is really hot, it is better for me to sit in the shade in a well-ventilated area, as getting too hot can increase the itching and soreness. It would be good if I could sit near to a fan or bring in my own fan.

- In the winter, the radiators can make me feel really hot and itchy too, so it is best if I can sit in the coolest area of the classroom.

- I don't sleep well at night when the itching is bad and medication can make me feel very tired the next day. Teachers need to understand that I am not being rude if I yawn in school. I really can't help it.

- Teachers need to keep an eye on me to make sure no one is being mean to me at school about my skin. It would be great to have someone I could go to talk to about this.

- When I was in primary school, it would have helped me to feel happier about my skin if my teachers had done some of the school activities suggested by the National Eczema Society so that my classmates could have understood more without me having to explain.

- Teachers need to understand how hard it is to write when my hands are cracked and bleeding.

- Teachers also need to understand how hard it is to concentrate on the lesson when my whole body is itching and I am trying so hard not to scratch.

- When my Eczema is particularly bad, it would be good if there was somewhere private that I could change for PE and go to put on some cream.

- School jumpers and blazers can be itchy and also make me overheat. It would be good if I didn't have to wear these all the time in hot weather or when school is warm inside in the winter.

- Sometimes exams and tests can make me feel really nervous and anxious (like many children), and this can really affect my Eczema. I may need to apply creams or to take antihistamines during the day to help.

- Sports, games and running around, especially when it is warm, can affect my skin and I may need to take regular breaks in the shade to cool down.

More information on the different treatments available for Eczema

BATH OILS

Having a warm bath each day is a good way to cleanse and moisturise the skin and to help keep infections at bay. Using a suitable bath oil or lotion will help add moisture to the skin and cleanse the skin. Never use bubble baths or soaps, as these will irritate the skin. Your doctor or pharmacist can recommend emollients that are suitable products for the bath. Gently pat the skin dry with a clean towel and immediately apply your emollients to lock in the skin's natural moisture and repair the skin's barrier.

STEROID CREAMS

These are also called topical corticosteroids (topical means "applied to the skin"). They are usually preparations made with a small percentage of the active ingredient in a base ointment, cream or gel. They work by reducing the inflammation and can be very effective at controlling flare-ups and allowing the skin to heal. Steroid creams in the UK come in different strengths: mild, moderate, potent and very potent.

The doctor will prescribe a suitable strength, depending on your age, how severe your Eczema is and where on your body your Eczema has flared. This is important to get your Eczema under control. Make sure to ask your doctor, nurse or pharmacist to explain where to apply the steroid cream, how often and how much to put on. You may be prescribed different strengths for different areas of the body, for example a mild strength for your face and a moderate or potent steroid for your body.

Long-term use of topical corticosteroids can have side effects, such as thinning of the skin, although with proper use, as directed by doctors and other health professionals, side effects should be minimal.

ANTIHISTAMINE TABLETS

Sedative antihistamines may help you to feel sleepy when the itch may otherwise keep you awake. The common antihistamines used for hayfever offer no benefit.

STEROID TABLETS

Oral steroids (corticosteroids) are only used when Eczema is very severe and not responding to other treatments. They can help by reducing inflammation and itching and are usually used for a short period to bring the Eczema under control again.

IMMUNE SUPPRESSANTS

As Atopic Eczema is triggered by an abnormal immune response, immune suppressant tablets and creams/ointments can help to dampen down this immune response. They help to reduce inflammation and redness. They are only used on people with severe Eczema when other therapies are not working. They may be applied to the skin, called topical calcineurin inhibitors, or they may be oral tablets – taken by mouth. If tablets are recommended they will be supervised by dermatologists and you will need to be referred to the local hospital.

PASTE BANDAGES

These can be used to moisturise and protect areas of Eczema on most parts of the body. They can contain calamine, coal tar, zinc or other emollients. Don't use bandages on infected skin.

WET-WRAPPING

Following a bath, a large amount of emollient is applied to the skin, and then a wet layer of tube bandage, followed by a dry layer. This can be an effective way of keeping the skin moist, cool and protected and feeling less itchy and more comfortable. The National Eczema Society has a booklet on wraps, paste bandages and therapeutic clothing, which includes a comprehensive guide to wet-wrapping.

ANTIBIOTICS

These can be prescribed to treat Eczema that is infected.

PHOTOTHERAPY

UVA and UVB light therapy is used in the treatment of Eczema.

PSYCHOLOGICAL THERAPY

Research has shown that cognitive behavioural therapy (CBT), relaxation therapy and meditation have all helped with the symptoms of Eczema.

Other health conditions related to Eczema

ASTHMA

Asthma is a common long-term lung condition that makes it hard to breathe properly. It can develop at any age, but you are more likely to have Asthma if a member of your family has it. Asthma symptoms can appear when certain triggers irritate the airways. Some common Asthma triggers are dust mites, pollen, fur, smoke, exercise and cold air. Chest infections can also make Asthma worse.

There isn't a cure for Asthma at the moment, but there are some good treatments to help control it.

For more information, see: www.asthma.org.uk. You may also find this book useful: Mills, L. *Can I tell you about Asthma? A guide for friends, family and professionals.* London: Jessica Kingsley Publishers (2012).

ALLERGIC RHINITIS (HAY FEVER)

Hay fever is mostly caused by an allergic reaction to things around us, such as pollen, dust mites, animal fur or feathers and moulds in damp places. These are called allergens.

Symptoms of hay fever may include: itchy, sore and watery eyes, blocked and itchy nose, sneezing, an itchy throat and inner ear and headaches. A person with hay fever may get all of the symptoms or only one or two.

When someone has an allergy, their body produces a chemical called histamine. If you have these symptoms you should talk to your pharmacist or GP and they may suggest a type of medicine called an antihistamine.

Read more here: www.allergyuk.org.

Recommended reading and organisations

BOOKS FOR YOUNGER CHILDREN

Hughes, J. (2012) *Emmy's Eczema (Dinosaur Friends)*. London: Wayland.

Leigh, J. (2013) *Rachel has Eczema (Dr Spot's Casebooks)*. London: Red Kite Books.

BOOKS FOR OLDER CHILDREN AND YOUNG PEOPLE

Chilman-Blair, K. and Rimmer, I. (2013) *Medikidz Explain Eczema: What's Up with Kenzie?* London: Medikidz Publishing.

Parker, V. (2011) *I Know Someone with Eczema (Young Explorer: Understanding Health Issues)*. Oxford: Raintree.

BOOKS FOR ADULTS

Charman, C. and Lawton, S. (2006) *Eczema: The Treatments and Therapies that Really Work*. London: Robinson Publishing.

Eckersley, J. (2007) *Living with Eczema*. London: SPCK Publishing.

Mitchell, T. and Hepplewhite, A. (2005) *Eczema ("At Your Fingertips" Guide)*. London: Class Publishing.

ORGANISATIONS

UK

British Association of Dermatologists
Willan House
4 Fitzroy Square
London
W1T 5HQ
Phone: 020 7383 0266
Fax: 020 7388 5263

Email: admin@bad.org.uk
Website: www.bad.org.uk

The British Association of Dermatologists is a charity whose charitable objectives are the practice, teaching, training and research of dermatology. It works with the Department of Health (DH), patient bodies and commissioners across the UK, advising on best practice and the provision of dermatology services across all service settings.

National Eczema Society
Hill House
Highgate Hill
London
N19 5NA
Phone: 0800 089 1122 (Monday to Friday, 8am to 8pm)
Email: helpline@eczema.org
Website: www.eczema.org

The National Eczema Society has two principal aims: first, to provide people with independent and practical advice about treating and managing Eczema, and, second, to raise awareness of the needs of those with Eczema with health-care professionals, teachers and the government in the UK.

USA

National Eczema Association
4460 Redwood Highway Suite 16D
San Rafael, CA 94903-1953
Phone: (1800)8187546 or (415)4993474
Email: info@nationaleczema.org
Website: http://nationaleczema.org

The National Eczema Association is striving to improve the quality of life for individuals with Eczema through research, support and education in the USA.

Canada

Eczema Society of Canada
411 The Queensway South
PO Box 25009
Keswick
Ontario
L4P 2C7
Phone: 1 855 ECZEMA 1
Website: www.eczemahelp.ca

The Eczema Society of Canada is a registered Canadian charity, dedicated to education Eczema awareness, providing support and supporting research.

Australia

Eczema Association of Australasia Inc
ABN 47 072 394 542
PO Box 1784 DC
Cleveland
QLD 4163
Phone: +61 7 32063633
Email: itchy@eczema.org.au
Website: http://eczema.org.au

The Eczema Association of Australasia's aim is to improve the life for those involved with Eczema through community representation and education.